HOW TO LOSE WEIGHT

TIPS FOR LOOSING WEIGHT WITHOUT DIET

CYRIL LAKES

Contents

CHAPTER ONE

INTRODUCTION

Changing your lifestyle to support healthy food, regular exercise, and positive behavior changes is the key to losing weight without resorting to traditional diets. This strategy, which aims for slow and long-lasting weight loss, places more emphasis on long-term behaviors than on temporary constraints. We'll look at practical methods and ideas in this book to help you lose weight without dieting, so you can increase your metabolism, make better decisions, and reach your goal weight in a long-term way. Together, we can go on this path towards a happier, healthier version of ourselves free from the limitations of restrictive diets.

Creating the scene: Weight loss without the need for typical dieting

Losing weight frequently evokes ideas of calorie tracking, tight diets, and suffering in today's health-conscious culture. It doesn't have to be this way, though. Not only is it feasible to lose weight without using standard diets, but the benefits may also be more long-lasting and durable.

Adopting a comprehensive strategy that stresses fueling your body, embracing regular physical activity, and making mindful lifestyle adjustments is vital, as opposed to relying only on band-aid solutions or dramatic methods. You can reach your weight loss objectives in a way that feels powerful and long-lasting by reorienting the focus from stringent regulations and limits to developing lifelong healthy behaviors.

We'll go over useful tactics, research-backed ideas, and doable advice in this book to help you shed pounds without using conventional dieting techniques. We'll explore the many facets of a holistic approach to weight loss that fosters general well-being and long-term success, from mindful eating and portion control to finding joy in physical activity and developing a positive mindset. Prepare to set out on a path to a better, more contented version of yourself, where self-care and enduring habits are prioritized.

The significance of adopting a sustainable lifestyle

Long-term weight loss and maintenance depend heavily on sustainable lifestyle adjustments. While quick cures and fad diets could produce short-term benefits, they frequently result in rebound weight gain and can be harmful to one's general health and wellbeing. Here's why making long-term lifestyle adjustments is crucial for effective weight loss:

Long-Term Success: Rather than depending on band-aid fixes, sustainable lifestyle modifications emphasize the development of lifelong healthy habits. You increase your chances of achieving long-term weight loss and avoiding weight gain by making small, sustainable modifications to your daily routine, food, and exercise regimen.

Better Health Outcomes: Long-term lifestyle adjustments boost general health and wellbeing in addition to aiding in weight loss. You may lower your chance of developing chronic illnesses like diabetes, heart disease, and some types of cancer by making self-care a priority, eating better, exercising more, and managing stress.

Balanced Approach: Sustainable lifestyle modifications encourage a balanced approach to eating and living, in contrast to restrictive diets that only concentrate on reducing calories or excluding whole food groups. This entails finding pleasure in engaging in enjoyable physical activity, eating a range of healthful foods in moderation, and practicing mindful eating.

Enhanced Metabolism: Excessive calorie restriction and crash diets can slow down your metabolism and cause muscle loss, which makes it more difficult to keep off weight over the long run. Conversely, sustainable lifestyle modifications help to maintain a healthy metabolism by giving your body the nourishment and energy it requires to perform at its best.

Good Relationship with Food and Body: Conventional dieting frequently results in emotions of guilt, deprivation, and anxiety related to food, which can have a detrimental effect on your relationship with food and how you feel about your body. A more positive and balanced approach to eating is encouraged by sustainable lifestyle changes, which also promote a healthier mindset and relationship with your body.

Enhanced Vitality and Energy: Making lasting lifestyle adjustments can boost vitality and energy levels while also enhancing mood. Overall health and quality of life are influenced by stress management, enough sleep, a balanced diet, and regular physical activity.

Preventing Weight Cycling: Often referred to as yo-yo dieting, weight cycling is the practice of people gradually losing and gaining weight. There may be detrimental impacts on one's physical and mental well-being from this pattern of weight fluctuations. Sustainable lifestyle adjustments encourage steady, moderate progress toward long-term weight control objectives, which helps break this pattern.

Making long-term lifestyle adjustments is crucial to losing weight successfully and maintaining it while also enhancing general health and wellbeing. Not only will you accomplish your weight loss objectives by concentrating on creating long-lasting healthy habits, but you'll also reap the many advantages of leading a well-rounded and satisfying life.

Recognizing the Fundamentals of Weight Loss

It's crucial to comprehend the fundamentals of weight loss in order to create tactics that will help you reach your objectives. While there are many variables that might affect weight reduction, such as genetics, metabolism, and health issues, there are basic guidelines that work for the majority of people. The following is a summary of important weight loss concepts:

Caloric Balance: Losing weight happens when your body gradually uses less calories than it takes in. As a result, there is a calorie deficit, which forces your body to burn fat that has been stored as fuel and causes weight reduction. On the other hand, weight gain results from consuming more calories than your body requires. Achieving and maintaining weight loss depends on knowing your calorie demands and modifying your intake accordingly.

Nutrient Density: Make an effort to eat meals high in nutrients, such as fiber, vitamins, and minerals, without adding too many calories. Fruits, vegetables, lean meats, whole grains, and healthy fats are examples of foods high in nutrients. In addition to promoting general health, these meals also help you feel satisfied for longer periods of time, which makes it simpler to control cravings and hunger while cutting calories.

Portion Control: To prevent overindulging, be careful of portion sizes and consume in moderation. Portion control is paying attention to serving sizes and your body's signals of hunger and fullness. You can maintain a healthy, balanced diet and control your calorie intake by eating nutrient-dense foods in smaller portions.

Balanced Macronutrients: To promote general health and satiety, include a healthy proportion of fats, proteins, and carbs in your diet. Energy comes from carbohydrates, growth and repair of muscles are supported by proteins, and hormone production and nutrition absorption are dependent on fats. Given your unique requirements and dietary preferences, try to consume a macronutrient distribution that is balanced.

Frequent Exercise: Include regular exercise in your regimen to boost energy expenditure, develop lean muscle mass, and aid in weight loss. For general health and weight control, aerobic exercise (such as walking, running, and cycling) and strength training (such as weightlifting, resistance training) are both crucial. Aim for 75 minutes of vigorous-intensity aerobic activity or at least 150 minutes of moderate-intensity aerobic activity per week, in addition to two or more days of muscle-strengthening activities.

Hydration: Throughout the day, make sure you drink lots of water to stay hydrated. Water boosts metabolism and lowers calorie intake, which may help with weight loss. It also supports a number of body processes and regulates hunger. Try to consume eight glasses of water or more if you live in a hot area or are physically active each day.

Prioritize getting a good night's sleep because getting too little sleep can mess with your hormones that control hunger, make you crave more high-calorie foods, and slow down your metabolism. To assist with weight loss and general well-being, set a regular sleep routine and aim for seven to nine hours of sleep each night.

Stress management: Reduce stress by engaging in deep breathing exercises, yoga, meditation, or mindfulness training. Prolonged stress can impede weight loss attempts by causing emotional eating, elevated cortisol levels (a stress hormone linked to weight gain), and irregular sleep habits.

You can create a thorough plan for reaching your weight loss objectives in a sustainable, healthy way by comprehending and putting these weight loss ideas into practice. Keep in mind that every person will react differently to food and exercise, so it's critical to determine the strategy that will work best for you and your particular requirements.

CHAPTER TWO

Practices of Mindful Eating

Without using harsh dieting techniques, mindful eating can be an effective strategy for encouraging weight loss. Through mindfulness of your body's signals of hunger and fullness, as well as your thoughts and feelings related to food, you may cultivate a more positive relationship with food and make more deliberate eating decisions. The following mindful eating techniques can be included into your regular routine:

Eat With Mindfulness: Take your time, enjoy every bite, and focus on the flavor, texture, and aroma of your food. When eating, stay away from devices like laptops, phones, and TVs so that you may give your whole attention to the meal.

Pay Attention to Your Body: Make sure your eating habits are guided by your body's indications of hunger and fullness. Rather than eating because you're bored, stressed out, or out of habit, eat when you're hungry and stop when you're satisfied. Check in with yourself before, during, and after meals to gauge your level of hunger and contentment. This is a mindful eating technique.

Select Nutrient-Dense Foods: Give your body the nourishment and long-lasting energy it needs by making nutrient-dense foods a priority. Make a point of including whole grains, lean meats, colorful fruits, veggies, healthy fats, and whole grains in your meals and snacks. Select meals that promote your general health and well-being and make you feel wonderful.

Exercise Portion Control: Pay attention to serving sizes and steer clear of excessive portions, particularly when dining out or consuming packaged foods. Measure cups, plates, or your own hand size as visual indicators to help you determine the right portion sizes and prevent overindulging.

Eat with Intention: Prior to starting to eat, stop, consider your motivations and the outcomes you want to achieve from the meal. Do you eat because you're bored, stressed out, or responding to something else emotionally? You can make more deliberate eating decisions that support your objectives and morals by becoming more aware of the reasons behind your eating habits.

Develop Gratitude: Give thanks for the food on your plate and the energy it gives your body. Whether the food was prepared at home or from a supermarket, pause to acknowledge the work that went into it. Developing an attitude of appreciation and thankfulness can improve eating experiences and promote a healthier connection with food.

Mindful Snacking: When choosing a snack, pay attention to your body's hunger signals and select wholesome foods that both satiate your cravings and advance your health objectives. Choose whole foods over manufactured snacks that are heavy in sugar, salt, or bad fats. Examples of these include fruits, vegetables, nuts, seeds, and yogurt.

Exercise Self-Compassion: When it comes to your eating habits, be gentle to yourself and exercise self-compassion. Adopt a nonjudgmental mindset toward others and yourself and refrain from having critical or judgmental thoughts about the foods you choose to eat. Recall that mindful eating is not about aiming for perfection when it comes to eating rather, it is about finding balance and enjoying it.

You may support your weight reduction objectives, create a better relationship with food, and change your eating habits by implementing mindful eating practices into your everyday routine instead of using severe or restrictive diets. Accept the benefits of mindfulness, pay attention to your body, and relish the feeling of feeding your body well-balanced, fulfilling meals.

Making Nutritious Food Selections

One of the most important things about losing weight without using conventional dieting techniques is choosing healthy foods. You may support your weight loss objectives and advance general health and well-being by putting an emphasis on providing your body with nutrient-dense foods and eating a balanced diet. Here are some pointers for selecting wholesome foods:

Make Whole Foods Your Top Priority: Opt for minimally processed, whole foods that are high in nutrients and devoid of artificial ingredients, bad fats, and added sugars. As the cornerstone of your diet, choose fruits, vegetables, whole grains, lean meats, and healthy fats.

Fill Up on Fiber: To encourage satiety and control hunger, include a lot of foods high in fiber in your meals and snacks. Fiber prolongs feelings of fullness, which lowers the risk of overeating and aids in weight loss. Fruits, vegetables, whole grains, legumes, nuts, and seeds are all excellent sources of fiber.

Choose Lean Proteins: To help with muscle growth, repair, and maintenance while keeping you feeling full, include lean protein sources in your meals. Pick lean meats like turkey, chicken, fish, and lean beef or pork chops. You can also choose plant-based protein sources like lentils, tofu, and tempeh.

Incorporate Healthy Fats: To promote general health and fullness, incorporate healthy fats into your diet. Don't be afraid of fat. Pick unsaturated fat-rich foods like avocados, almonds, seeds, olive oil, and fatty seafood like sardines and salmon. These fats help to keep you feeling full and content while supplying vital nutrients and supporting heart health.

Reduce Added Sugar Intake: Add as little as possible to your diet to avoid adding unnecessary calories that don't offer any nutritional benefit. Watch out for hidden sugar sources in processed foods, sugar-filled drinks, snacks, and desserts. Instead, use naturally sweet things like fruits or tiny amounts of dark chocolate to sate your sweet desire.

Watch Portion Sizes: Be mindful of portion sizes and steer clear of excessive amounts, particularly when consuming packaged or restaurant-style food. Measure cups, plates, or your own hand size as visual indicators to help you determine the right portion sizes and prevent overindulging.

Keep Yourself Hydrated: To stay hydrated and promote general health and weight loss efforts, sip lots of water throughout the day. Water keeps your body operating at its best, controls hunger, and removes pollutants. Try to consume eight glasses of water or more if you live in a hot area or are physically active each day.

Practice Mindful Eating: Recognize your eating patterns and use your body's signals of hunger and fullness to help you make informed food decisions. To prevent overeating, take your time eating, enjoy every meal, and pay attention to your body's cues. Enjoying the tastes, textures, and scents of your meal should take precedence over counting calories in a mindless manner.

Plan and Prepare Meals: To encourage good eating practices throughout the week, set aside time to plan and prepare balanced meals and snacks in advance. Prepare meals ahead of time, stock your kitchen with wholesome items, and prepare wholesome snacks for when hunger strikes.

Permit Flexibility: Adopt a flexible eating strategy that keeps the emphasis on general balance and moderation but permits special occasions and indulgences. Steer clear of categorizing things as "good" or "bad" and strive for a balanced diet that nourishes your body and mind.

You may support your weight loss objectives while nourishing your body and advancing general health and well-being by choosing foods wisely and giving priority to those high in nutrients. To develop a long-lasting eating strategy that promotes your long-term health and happiness, put your attention on combining complete foods, balancing macronutrients, and paying attention to your body's hunger and fullness cues.

Creating Balanced Meals

Creating balanced meals is essential to losing weight without using conventional dieting techniques. You can support your weight loss objectives while making sure your body gets the vital nutrients it needs to flourish by including a range of nutrient-dense foods in your meals and paying attention to portion control. How to prepare meals that are balanced to help you lose weight?

Lean Proteins: To help you feel full and to support the growth and repair of your muscles, start by including a lean source of protein in each meal. Select from items like beans, lentils, tofu, tempeh, skinless chicken, fish, and low-fat dairy. Aim for 25% of your plate to be made up of items high in protein.

Add Colorful veggies: To enhance fiber consumption, encourage satiety, and supply vital vitamins and minerals, cover half of your plate with a range of colorful veggies. To enhance taste, texture, and nutritional value of your meals, incorporate a variety of leafy greens, cruciferous vegetables, peppers, tomatoes, carrots, cucumbers, and other non-starchy veggies.

Include Whole Grains: To supply complex carbs and long-lasting energy, include a dish of whole grains or starchy vegetables in your diet. Select foods like corn, oats, sweet potatoes, barley, bulgur, brown rice, quinoa, and whole wheat pasta. Aim to have starchy veggies or whole grains make up around a quarter of your plate.

Add Good Fats: To increase nutrient absorption, boost cognitive function, and encourage satiety, include sources of good fats in your meals. Add avocado, nuts, seeds, olives, olive oil, flaxseed, chia seeds, and fatty fish like trout, salmon, or mackerel to the list of alternatives. Small amounts of healthy fats can be used as toppings or for cooking to give your food more taste and texture.

Don't Forget Fiber: To assist weight loss efforts, maintain blood sugar levels, and improve digestive health, make sure your meals are full of foods high in fiber. To add texture and bulk to your meals, include sources of fiber such beans, lentils, fruits, nuts, and seeds along with veggies and whole grains.

Watch Portion proportions: Be mindful of portion proportions and steer clear of excessive servings, particularly for high-calorie items like grains, nuts, and oils. Measure cups, plates, or your own hand size as visual indicators to help you determine the right portion sizes and prevent overindulging. To prevent consuming too many calories, be aware of portion distortion and serve yourself lesser quantities.

Remain Hydrated: To promote healthy digestion, metabolism, and general well-being, remember to stay hydrated throughout the day with water or other calorie-free liquids. When consuming meals and snacks, try to stay hydrated and avoid dehydration, which can occasionally be confused with hunger.

Balance Your Plate: For long-lasting energy and satisfaction, try to prepare meals that are well-balanced that contain a variety of proteins, carbs, and healthy fats. Try blending various ingredients and flavors to make filling and healthy meals that will help you reach your weight loss objectives.

You may create balanced meals that promote weight reduction without turning to restrictive dieting techniques by including lean proteins, vibrant veggies, whole grains, healthy fats, and foods high in fiber in your meals. You may also remember to control portion sizes and drink enough of water. Make an effort to prepare filling meals that promote your general health and well-being and fuel your activities by consuming foods high in nutrients.

The Importance of Hydration for Managing Weight

One of the most important components of losing weight without resorting to typical dieting techniques is staying hydrated, which is also critical for weight control and general health. Maintaining proper hydration is beneficial for several body processes, such as digestion, metabolism, and hunger control. Here are some suggestions for including water in your weight loss strategy as well as how it affects weight management:

Appetite Regulation: Having a glass of water prior to meals will help curb hunger and increase feelings of fullness, which can help cut back on calories and aid in weight loss. Water consumption prior to meals is associated with a lower total calorie intake, according to studies, which makes it a useful tactic for controlling appetite and portion sizes.

Boost Your Metabolism: Drinking enough water helps your body's metabolism, which makes it easier for it to turn food into energy. Adequate hydration helps sustain metabolic rate and optimizes burning of calories; dehydration can slow down metabolism and impede weight loss efforts. Water consumption throughout the day can improve weight management by maintaining a healthy metabolism.

Calorie-Free Hydration: Water is calorie-free and delivers hydration without adding extra calories to your diet, in contrast to sugary drinks like soda, juice, or energy drinks. By avoiding liquid calories from beverages that might cause weight gain, choosing water as your main beverage helps lower overall calorie intake and promote weight loss.

Fluid Balance: Drinking enough water keeps the body's fluid balance, which is necessary for the best possible health for all of the body's tissues, cells, and organs. Dehydration can cause bloating and water retention, which can make you feel uneasy and heavier. Maintaining proper hydration can help maintain fluid balance, lessen bloating, and result in a more comfortable, leaner physique.

Exercise Performance: For the best possible exercise performance, endurance, and recuperation, hydration is essential. You may perform better during exercises and burn more calories by drinking adequate water before, during, and after exercise. It also helps to prevent dehydration, maintain electrolyte balance, and support energy levels.

Hunger vs. Thirst: Occasionally, people confuse their emotions of thirst for hunger, which causes them to overindulge in calories. Drinking enough water during the day will help you recognize the difference between hunger and thirst signals, which will stop you from overeating and aid in your weight loss attempts. To stay hydrated and prevent mindless munching, always have a water bottle on hand and sip on water frequently.

Drinking water throughout the day is a good way to stay hydrated. Start with a glass of water in the morning and continue with sipping water with meals and snacks. Always carry a water bottle to remind yourself to stay hydrated and drink often. To enhance taste without adding extra calories, add a hint of lemon, cucumber, or mint to your water.

Track Your Hydration Level: Be alert for indications of dehydration, such as headaches, lethargy, dark urine, or dry mouth, and make drinking water your first priority to avoid these problems. Try to maintain a pale yellow urine color, which indicates proper hydration, by drinking enough water. To stay hydrated, pay attention to your body's thirst cues and sip water whenever you feel it coming on.

It is possible to enhance appetite regulation, metabolism, exercise performance, and general health while supporting successful weight management by making hydration a priority and implementing it into your weight reduction strategy. Instead of using conventional dieting techniques to assist your weight loss goals, make drinking water a habit, pay attention to your body's thirst signals, and keep hydrated throughout the day.

Making physical activity a priority is crucial to losing weight without resorting to conventional dieting techniques. Frequent exercise aids sustainable weight management, increases metabolism, and improves general health in addition to burning calories. Here's how to make exercise a priority when trying to lose weight:

Select Physical Activities You Love: Look for physical activities that you actually look forward to engaging in. Choosing activities you enjoy enhances the likelihood that you will keep with them over time, whether it's walking, jogging, swimming, cycling, dancing, or playing sports.

Try out a variety of things until you discover ones that you enjoy.

Set Achievable and practical Fitness objectives: Based on your hobbies, lifestyle, and present level of fitness, set attainable and practical fitness objectives. Setting clear, quantifiable objectives keeps you motivated and accountable, whether your goals are to increase your daily step count, work out for a specified amount of time each week, or learn a new exercise method.

Mix It Up: To keep things fresh and avoid monotony, mix up your training regimen with a range of exercises and activities. To improve total fitness and target different muscle groups, incorporate functional motions, strength training, aerobic activities, and flexibility exercises.

Changing up your regimen also keeps your body from plateauing and exposes it to new difficulties.

Put Consistency First: Schedule regular workouts and try your best to keep to them to make physical activity a non-negotiable part of your daily routine. Instead of striving for perfection, focus on consistency, and be willing to modify your workout regimen to account for alterations in your schedule or personal circumstances. Daily activity, even brief bursts, build up and support overall fitness and calorie burning.

Look for Opportunities to Move: Make an effort to move more throughout your day by walking or biking for errands, gardening, performing housework, or using the stairs rather than the elevator. Increasing your everyday physical activity level assists weight loss attempts without the need for specific workout sessions. It also helps to increase calorie expenditure.

Emphasis on Non-Exercise Activity: Prioritize NEAT (Non-Exercise Activity Thermogenesis), or non-exercise physical activity, in addition to scheduled workouts. NEAT includes the number of calories burned from routine tasks like standing, walking, fidgeting, and housework. Elevating NEAT levels can have a major effect on overall energy expenditure and facilitate weight loss in the absence of structured exercise.

Progress Gradually: As your fitness level rises, start at a comfortable intensity level and progressively raise the length, frequency, and intensity of your workouts.

CHAPTER THREE

Pay attention to your body and try not to overextend yourself, particularly if you're just starting out or coming back to the gym after a hiatus. Gradual growth guarantees long-term sustainability and aids in injury prevention.

Make It Social: To increase social support and accountability for your fitness program, work out with friends, family, or fellow fitness enthusiasts. To meet people who have similar interests and aspirations, sign up for community workout programs, sports teams, or group fitness courses. Exercise can be more motivating and pleasurable when you have a support network.

Make Recovery Your Top Priority: To avoid burnout, lower your chance of injury, and encourage muscle growth and regeneration, give yourself enough time to rest and recuperate in between sessions. To enhance recovery and general well-being, include rest days in your schedule, change up the length and intensity of your exercises, and place a high priority on rest, diet, and stress reduction.

Track Your Progress: To keep yourself inspired and goal-focused, keep an eye on your progress and acknowledge your accomplishments along the way. Maintain a fitness log, track your exercises, steps, and other metrics using a wearable or fitness app, and recognize and acknowledge your accomplishments when you reach new heights in your strength, endurance, or general fitness.

Without using conventional dieting techniques, you may promote weight loss, improve general health, and improve your quality of life by making physical activity a priority and a regular part of your daily. To develop an exercise regimen that is sustainable and effective for you, choose activities you enjoy, make realistic goals, place a high value on consistency, and pay attention to what your body needs.

Controlling Stress and Emotional Consumption

To lose weight without using conventional dieting techniques, emotional eating and stress management are essential. Your attempts to lose weight can be hampered by stress and emotions, which can also lead to overeating and cravings for unhealthy foods. The following techniques can assist you in efficiently managing stress and emotional eating:

Determine Triggers: Keep an eye out for circumstances, feelings, or occasions that set off episodes of stress eating or emotional eating. Work deadlines, interpersonal disputes, boredom, loneliness, or depressive or anxious sensations are examples of common causes. Finding your triggers will help you create more effective techniques to deal with them.

Use Stress Management tactics: To lower stress levels and stop emotional eating, incorporate stress management tactics into your everyday routine. Stress hormones can be lowered and relaxation can be encouraged via methods including progressive muscle relaxation, yoga, meditation, deep breathing, and mindfulness.

Find Healthy Coping Mechanisms: Instead of turning to food for solace and release, consider healthy coping strategies to replace emotional eating. Take part in soul-nourishing and calming activities, such taking a stroll in the outdoors, writing in a notebook, listening to music, taking up a hobby, spending time with loved ones, or getting help from a therapist or counselor.

Develop Mindful Eating: Rather than eating in reaction to feelings or outside stimuli, pay attention to your body's physical signs of hunger and fullness. When deciding when you're genuinely hungry and content, take your time, enjoy every piece, chew your meal well, and pay attention to your body's cues.

Maintain a Food Journal: Monitor your eating habits, feelings, and situations that lead to emotional eating by keeping a food journal. You can spot patterns, obtain understanding of your eating habits, and make more deliberate decisions going forward by keeping a journal of what you eat, when you eat, and how you feel both before and after.

Establish a Support System: Encircle yourself with friends, family, or a support group that will be there for you while you lose weight to offer accountability, understanding, and encouragement. Talk to people about your challenges and accomplishments, and ask for help if you're anxious or inclined to overindulge in food for emotional reasons.

Practice Self-Compassion: When you encounter obstacles or disappointments, remember to treat yourself with kindness and self-compassion. Refrain from criticizing or blaming yourself for emotional eating episodes; instead, put your attention on resilience, forgiveness, and self-care. Remind yourself that mistakes are normal and part of the path since you are human.

Address Underlying Issues: If your attempts to control your stress and emotions are not enough to stop emotional eating, you may need to seek professional assistance to address underlying emotional or psychological problems. Healthy coping methods and effective tools for overcoming emotional eating can be developed through therapy, counseling, or support groups.

Distract Yourself: Find other tasks to occupy your time that will divert your attention from eating when you are tempted to overindulge emotionally. To clear your head and focus, read a book, make a phone call, go for a stroll, listen to music, or take up a hobby.

Adopt a Moderation-Not-Deprivation mentality by letting yourself indulge in your favorite foods in moderation without feeling guilty or constrained. Restricting your intake of a certain meal can backfire, causing cravings and episodes of binge eating. Rather, concentrate on moderation, balance, and mindfully and joyfully including a range of foods into your diet.

Instead of using conventional dieting techniques, you can effectively manage stress and emotional eating while supporting your weight loss objectives by putting these tactics into practice and engaging in self-awareness, self-care, and self-compassion exercises. As you travel the path to a better, more fulfilled life and a healthy relationship with food, keep in mind that change takes time and practice self-compassion.

Obtaining Enough Rest

To lose weight without resorting to conventional dieting techniques, getting enough sleep is essential. Sleep is essential for controlling metabolism, hunger, energy levels, and general wellness. Sleep deprivation can interfere with hormone balance, heighten food cravings, and undermine attempts to lose weight. Here's how putting sleep first can help you achieve your weight loss objectives:

Controls Hunger Hormones: Sleeping enough sleep aids in the regulation of the hunger- and appetite-controlling hormones, ghrelin and leptin. These hormones are disturbed by sleep deprivation, which increases appetite and causes desires for high-calorie foods and overeating.

Making sleep a priority lowers the chance of overeating and aids in the maintenance of a healthy hormone balance.

Enhances Metabolism: Getting enough sleep promotes energy expenditure and metabolic processes, which makes it possible for your body to burn calories more effectively. On the other hand, a lack of sleep can impede metabolism and increase body weight. Getting enough sleep guarantees that your body's metabolism functions at their best, which promotes weight reduction and general well-being.

Lowers Stress and Cortisol Levels: Sleep has a critical role in stress management and the reduction of cortisol, a stress hormone linked to weight gain and the storage of fat in the abdomen. Prolonged sleep deprivation can cause stress, raised cortisol levels, and an increase in comfort food desires. Making sleep a priority lowers cortisol levels, eases stress, and promotes better eating practices.

Encourages Physical Activity: Getting enough sleep improves motivation, energy levels, and physical performance, which makes it simpler to work out regularly. A well-rested body is more likely to support weight loss efforts by increasing calorie expenditure. It also makes you feel more inspired and eager to incorporate movement into your daily routine.

Enhances Willpower and Decision-Making: Lack of sleep affects one's ability to think clearly, make decisions, and regulate impulses, which makes it more difficult to resist cravings and choose healthful foods. Making sleep a priority strengthens your willpower, sharpens your mind, and empowers you to make more deliberate decisions that support your weight reduction objectives.

Improves Muscle Growth and Recovery: Getting enough sleep is crucial for the growth, healing, and repair of muscles, particularly after physical activity or exercise. The body goes through several critical healing processes while you sleep, such as protein synthesis and muscular tissue restoration. Sleeping enough aids in muscle regeneration, lessens soreness in the muscles, and increases lean muscle mass—all of which raise metabolic rate and improve efficiency of weight reduction.

Creates Healthy Habits: Making sleep a priority is essential to general health and wellbeing and lays the groundwork for embracing other healthy lifestyle practices that aid in weight loss. Prioritizing sleep increases your likelihood of making better decisions during the day, such as eating a balanced diet, exercising, and effectively handling stress.

Provide a Sleep-Friendly Environment: Make sure your room is quiet, dark, and cold, and that your mattress and pillows are comfy to help you get a good night's sleep. Avoid staring at screens (such as phones, laptops, and TVs) right before bed since the blue light they emit might interfere with the generation of melatonin and cause sleep disturbances.

Adhere to a Regular Sleep Schedule: Even on weekends, keep a regular sleep schedule by going to bed and waking up at the same times every day. Over time, consistency enables your body's internal clock to stabilize and enhances the quality of your sleep. Depending on your own needs, try to get between seven and nine hours of sleep every night.

Practice Relaxation Techniques: To encourage sound sleep and lower stress levels, include relaxation techniques in your nightly routine. You may assist your body get ready for sleep by doing things like deep breathing exercises, reading, stretching gently, or practicing meditation.

Without turning to conventional dieting techniques, you can promote weight loss, enhance general health, and improve your well-being by making sleep a priority and making sure you get enough good sleep every night. Enjoy the many advantages that getting enough sleep provides for your body and mind by making it an indisputable part of your self-care regimen.

Establishing a Helpful Environment

To lose weight without using conventional dieting techniques, it is imperative to create a supportive environment. Your house, location of employment, social network, and daily schedule all have a big impact on how you eat, how active you are, and how you choose to live your life. The following techniques can be used to establish a welcoming atmosphere that encourages good behaviors and speeds up weight loss:

Encircle Yourself with Supportive People: Encircle yourself with people who support and encourage you in your weight loss efforts, such as friends, family, or a support group. Talk about your experience with people who can relate to your struggles and offer support, accountability, and inspiration as you go. Steer clear of people who try to undermine you or impede your growth.

Share Your Intentions and Goals: Let everyone know about your plans to lose weight, including your friends, family, and coworkers. Tell them how they can help you, whether it's by encouraging you, participating with you in healthful activities, or honoring your dietary decisions. Transparent communication promotes comprehension and establishes a nurturing atmosphere for your own journey.

Establish a Healthy Home Environment by putting wholesome snacks and foods in your kitchen that support your weight loss objectives. To prevent temptation and encourage healthier choices, keep harmful foods hidden from view or removed from the house. Organize your pantry and kitchen to increase the accessibility and convenience of nutritious options.

Meal Prep and Planning: Set aside time each week to prepare meals and make advance meal plans. To ensure easy access throughout the week, prepare nutritious meals and snacks ahead of time, portion them into individual containers, and keep them in the freezer or refrigerator. Making a meal plan for the week helps you avoid making rash judgments when you're hungry.

Set Yourself Up for Success at Work: Bring wholesome meals and snacks from home, pack a lunchbox or cooler with wholesome options, and restock your desk or workplace with wholesome snacks like yogurt, fruits, and nuts to foster a supportive work environment. To reduce temptation, don't have unhealthy snacks in your workspace.

Integrate Physical Activity into Your Environment: By integrating physical activity into your surroundings, you may make it a natural part of your everyday routine. Opt for active modes of transportation like walking or biking, use the stairs rather than the elevator, and plan to take regular breaks or meetings for walks. Make your home an exercise-friendly place by designating a room for exercise and having equipment close at hand.

Establish Routines and Healthy behaviors Together: Get your family or other home members involved in developing routines and healthy behaviors. As a family, plan and cook meals, include kids in grocery shopping and meal preparation, and spend time together doing physical activities or going outside. Prioritizing health within the family creates a supportive atmosphere and provides a good example for others.

Practice Stress Management and Self-Care: To enhance your general well-being and weight loss endeavors, give priority to stress management and self-care techniques. Include stress-relieving and relaxation-promoting pursuits including yoga, meditation, relaxation techniques, and hobbies. Maintaining your mental and emotional well-being helps create an atmosphere that is conducive to losing weight.

Seek Professional Assistance: If you're having trouble losing weight, think about getting help from healthcare experts like therapists, registered dietitians, personal trainers, or nutritionists. They can offer you individualized counsel, accountability, and encouragement. Gaining expert assistance can assist you in overcoming difficulties, navigating hurdles, and achieving long-term success.

Celebrate Your Progress and Milestones: To recognize your accomplishments and maintain motivation, celebrate your progress and milestones along the way. Whether it's hitting a weight reduction milestone, developing a new healthy habit, or completing a fitness objective, give yourself a pat on the back and acknowledge the progress you've achieved.

Instead of using conventional dieting techniques, you can develop healthy habits, get beyond challenges, and achieve long-term success by establishing a supportive atmosphere that supports your weight loss objectives. Be in the company of encouraging people, position yourself for success at work and at home, give self-care first priority, and, if necessary, seek professional advice. You may make long-lasting lifestyle adjustments that enhance happiness, health, and well-being if you have the correct surroundings and support network in place.

Monitoring Development and Modifying Approaches

It is vital to monitor weight reduction progress and modify tactics to get weight loss without turning to conventional dieting techniques. By keeping an eye on your progress, you may evaluate the success of your efforts, spot areas for development, and make the required corrections to keep moving in the direction of your objectives. Here's how to successfully monitor your progress and modify your methods in order to lose weight:

Establish Specific, Achievable Goals: To begin your weight loss journey, clearly define your goals. Having specific goals gives your efforts focus and incentive, whether your goals are to adopt healthier lifestyle choices, improve fitness levels, or lose a specific amount of weight.

Choose Your Tracking Methods: Depending on your goals, preferences, and way of life, choose the tracking techniques that are most effective for you. Keeping a food journal, monitoring exercise and physical activity, tracking body measures (waist circumference, body fat percentage, and weight), and using fitness applications or wearable technology to measure improvement are common tracking techniques.

Track Food Intake: If you'd like, make a note of everything you eat each day, including meals, snacks, serving sizes, and calorie counts. Be mindful of the kinds of food you're eating and the patterns and behaviors you follow when it comes to eating. By keeping track of your food consumption, you can become more conscious of your eating habits, pinpoint areas for development, and make necessary adjustments to promote weight loss.

Monitor Physical Activity: Keep tabs on your workout regimen and level of physical activity to make sure you're reaching your weekly activity targets. Maintain a journal of your workouts, noting the kind of activity, length, level of intensity, and frequency. Tracking your physical activity enables you to evaluate your development, spot patterns, and modify your training regimen as necessary to get the best effects.

Measure Body Composition: To monitor changes over time, take regular measurements of important body composition markers like weight, body fat percentage, and waist circumference. Make regular check-ins and use consistent measurement techniques to evaluate progress and modify your strategies as needed.

Celebrate non-scale victories and other progress indicators besides the scale number by keeping track of them. Observe improvements in your overall well-being, energy levels, mood, sleep quality, fitness level, and how well your clothes fit. These non-scale successes give you insightful feedback and inspire you to keep going.

Assess Progress Regularly: Schedule regular check-ins to assess your progress and analyze your monitoring data. Whether it's weekly, bi-weekly, or monthly, consistency is crucial to correctly assessing progress and making modifications as needed. Use this opportunity to reflect on your achievements, identify obstacles, and adapt your plans accordingly.

find Patterns and Trends: Examine your tracking information to find trends, patterns, and links between your actions and results. Look for factors such as eating habits, exercise routine, quality of sleep, stress levels, and hormone fluctuations that can be affecting your results. Finding patterns enables you to focus on problem areas and make focused changes to maximize outcomes.

Make Modifications Gradually: Modify your diet, exercise regimen, and lifestyle tactics as necessary in light of your tracking results and development. Instead of making big, abrupt changes at first, start small and make gradual improvements to increase sustainability and prevent overload. As you advance, keep an eye on how changes are impacting things and keep improving your strategy.

Remain Adaptive and Flexible: Adjust your tactics in response to your changing requirements, tastes, and situations. Losing weight is a dynamic process that may call for modifications along the road. Accept trial and error, grow from failures, and never give up on figuring out what will ultimately work best for you.

Without using conventional dieting techniques, you can successfully manage your weight reduction journey by keeping track of your progress, keeping an eye on important indications, and modifying your strategy in response to feedback. Maintain consistency, accountability, and commitment to your objectives, understanding that every little change will get you one step closer to long-term success.

Overcoming A Plateausis in Weight Loss

One of the most frequent obstacles to losing weight without resorting to conventional dieting techniques is getting beyond weight loss plateaus. When you reach a plateau in your weight loss attempts, it can be discouraging and upsetting because your progress is stopped. Still, there are a few tactics you can use to overcome obstacles and keep moving closer to your objectives:

Reevaluate Your Calorie Intake: Your calorie requirements may fluctuate in tandem with weight fluctuations. Make sure you're still in a calorie deficit if you've reached a plateau by reviewing your calorie intake. To accelerate weight loss, monitor your food consumption and think about reducing your calorie intake or changing the portions you eat.

Examine Your Food Selections: Consider your food selections more carefully and assess the caliber of your diet. Concentrate on eating full, nutrient-dense foods that promote satiety and general wellness. Prioritize lean proteins, fruits, vegetables, whole grains, and healthy fats while reducing your intake of processed foods, sugary snacks, and calorically-rich beverages.

Adjust the amount of protein, carbs, and fats in your diet to see if it helps you break through the plateau. Play around with your macronutrient ratios. While some people may respond better to changes in their intake of fat or carbohydrates, others may benefit more from an increase in protein to enhance muscle retention and metabolism.

Include More Physical exercise: To enhance calorie burning and promote weight loss, up your degree of physical exercise. You can include more cardio, strength, or high-intensity interval training (HIIT) sessions in your regimen, or you can just lengthen or intensify the workouts you already do. To overcome plateaus, put your attention on pushing yourself and going beyond of your comfort zone.

Modify Your Workout program: Add new movements, pursuits, or training techniques to your program to make it more interesting. Use a variety of exercise routines, such as circuit training, interval training, or outdoor exercises, to keep your body from becoming accustomed to one particular style of training. In addition to keeping you from becoming bored, cross-training works numerous muscle groups and increases your metabolism.

Boost Non-Exercise Activity: To increase total calorie expenditure, up your non-exercise physical activity, or NEAT (Non-Exercise Activity Thermogenesis). Seek out ways to increase your everyday physical activity, such as using the stairs, choosing to walk or bike instead of drive, standing up more often, and introducing movement into your regular tasks.

Set priorities. Stress and Sleep: Both your stress levels and the quality of your sleep might affect how quickly you lose weight. Try to get between seven and nine hours of good sleep every night to help with healing, metabolism, and hormone balance. Reduce cortisol levels and encourage relaxation by engaging in stress-reduction practices like deep breathing, yoga, mindfulness, and meditation.

Maintain Adequate Hydration: Make sure you are getting enough water throughout the day. Sometimes, dehydration can pass for hunger, which can result in overindulgence or cravings. Water consumption boosts metabolism, facilitates satiety, and facilitates digestion all of which are factors in weight loss.

Control Your Expectations and Show Patience: Recognize that weight reduction plateaus are a natural part of the process and do not indicate a lack of success. Have patience with yourself and have faith in the process; you will eventually see rewards from your persistence and consistency. Instead of getting fixated on short-term swings in the scale, concentrate on adopting durable lifestyle improvements.

Seek Support and Accountability: If you're having trouble breaking through a weight loss plateau, don't be afraid to ask friends, family, or a healthcare provider for help. Accountability and support from others can give you the drive and perspective you need to stay on course and overcome obstacles.

You may get over weight loss plateaus and keep moving in the direction of your target weight without using conventional dieting techniques by putting these suggestions into practice and being dedicated to your objectives. Celebrate every little accomplishment along the road and keep in mind that long-term success requires consistency, patience, and tenacity.

CONCLUSION

In conclusion, sustained lifestyle adjustments that put an emphasis on general health and well-being can help people lose weight without the need for traditional dieting techniques. You can get long-lasting weight loss and enhance your quality of life by putting an emphasis on providing your body with nutrient-dense foods, remaining physically active, controlling stress, getting enough sleep, and setting up a supportive atmosphere.

Adopting a balanced approach to exercise and nutrition instead of restrictive diets or fast fixes encourages long-term success and maintenance of a healthy weight. Adopt mindful eating techniques, choose wholesome foods, and plan meals that are balanced and meet your energy requirements and fitness goals.

Make regular physical activity a part of your schedule by mixing aerobic, weightlifting, flexibility, and enjoyable activities that will keep you engaged and motivated. Make time for self-care, stress relief, and enough sleep to improve overall health and maximize weight loss.

Keep in mind that growth might not always be linear and that obstacles like plateaus or setbacks are common parts of the journey. Remember that every little step you take toward your goals will bring you one step closer to your desired results, so be patient, persistent, and goal-focused.

Above all, remember that losing weight is a journey that involves not just physical adjustments but also behavioral, mental, and emotional enhancements. Throughout the process, keep an optimistic mindset, acknowledge and appreciate your successes, and practice self-compassion.

You can achieve long-term weight loss without using restrictive dieting techniques by adopting a lifestyle focused on wellness, equilibrium, and self-care. Have faith in your ability to transform your life, and relish the process of becoming a better, happier version of yourself.

THE END